JUICING RECIPES FOR GASTROPARESIS

Delicious Recipes to Soothe Your Stomach and Revitalize Your Health.

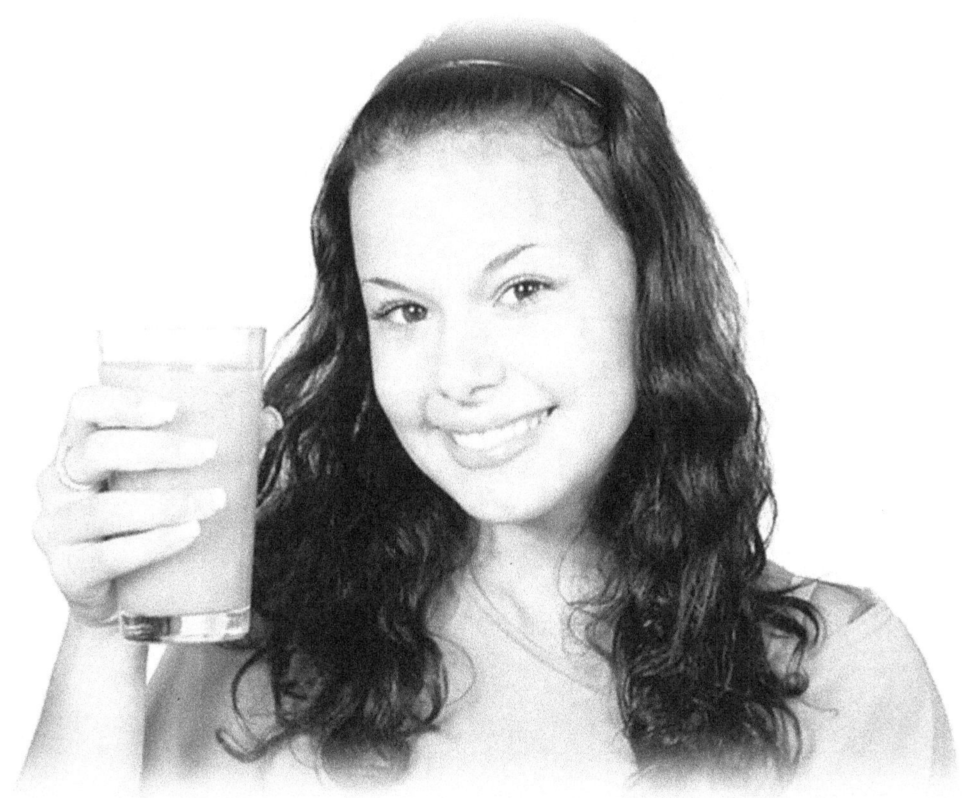

CHRISTIANA WHITE

GAIN ACCESS TO MORE BOOKS

DISCLAIMER

The recipes in this cookbook are provided for informational purposes only and are not intended as medical or professional advice. While the author and publisher have made every effort to ensure the accuracy and effectiveness of the recipes, they are not responsible for any adverse effects or consequences resulting from the use of the suggestions herein.

The information in this cookbook should not replace professional advice. Readers are advised to consult a healthcare provider or a culinary professional before making any significant changes to their diet or cooking practices.

Nutritional information is approximate and should be used as a guide only. Variations may occur due to product availability, food preparation, portion size, and other factors.

The author and publisher disclaim any liability in connection with the use of this information. It is the reader's responsibility to determine the value and quality of any recipe or instructions provided for food preparation and to determine the nutritional adequacy of the food to be consumed.

ABOUT THE AUTHOR

When it comes to tasty and nutritious cookbooks that turn wellness into a delightful journey, Christiana White is the author you turn to. She approaches cooking from a new angle and has a passion for creating wholesome food.

Motivated by her own pursuit of health, Christiana's books on Amazon are brimming with delectable recipes that demonstrate that eating healthily can be both simple and enjoyable. Her creative method makes cooking approachable to all skill levels by fusing entire, simple foods with flavors from around the world.

Readers of Christiana's meals gush about the beneficial effects her foods have on their lives outside of the kitchen. Her books are more than just recipes; they're guides for a happier, better way of life, resulting in everything from more energy to a revitalized passion for cooking.

Come along with Christiana to discover how to turn your meals into satisfying and joyful experiences. Discover the delightful intersection of health and flavor by delving into the colourful world of her cookbooks.

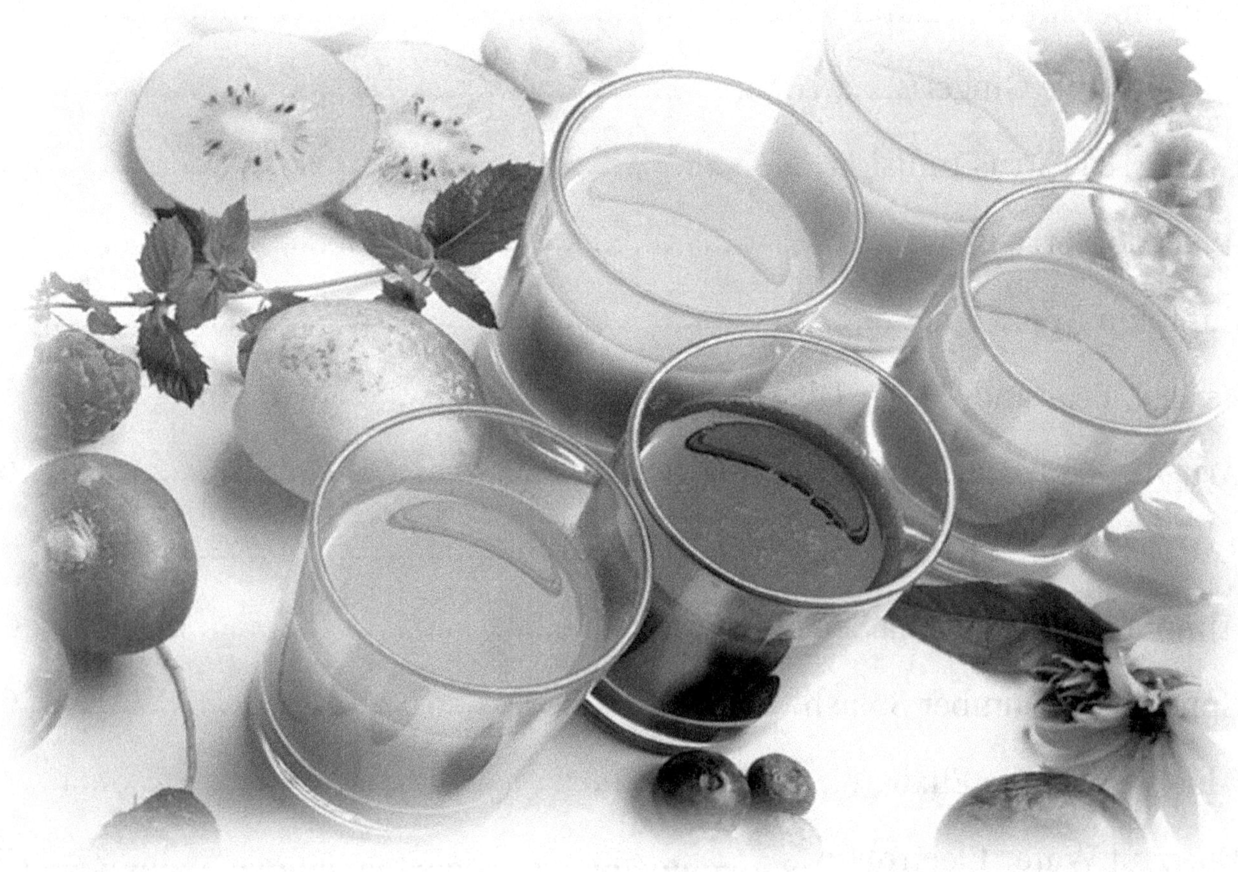

INTRODUCTION TO JUICING FOR GASTROPARESIS.

Welcome to "Juicing Recipes for Gastroparesis," a collection of nutritious and delicious juices created with your health in mind. If you are reading this, you may be all too familiar with the daily hardships that gastroparesis presents.

The ongoing hunt for foods that do not cause symptoms, as well as the fight to maintain a balanced diet, can be exhausting. However, these pages provide both hope and flavor in equal measure.

My experience with gastroparesis began with a close friend's diagnosis. Watching their struggle prompted me to discover a method to bring joy back into their meals. That's when I discovered the magic of juicing—a way to experience a wide range of Flavors without overpowering the digestive system.

This book is more than simply a compilation of recipes; it's a guide to navigating your nutritional needs with confidence. Each recipe has been meticulously created to guarantee that it is both safe for persons with gastroparesis and delicious to the taste.

From the cool "Cucumber Mint Cleanse" to the sweet "Papaya Peach Sip," there's a juice for every taste and occasion.

As someone who has spent years studying nutrition and working with gastroenterologists, I've designed these recipes to be soft on your stomach while yet giving the nutrients you require. You'll also find useful tips on juicing practices, symptom management, and getting the most of every cup.

So, whether you're new to gastroparesis or a seasoned master seeking for new ideas, this book will guide you through a world of flavor that's both safe and gratifying. Turn the page and let's go on this journey together. Your taste buds and stomach will appreciate you.

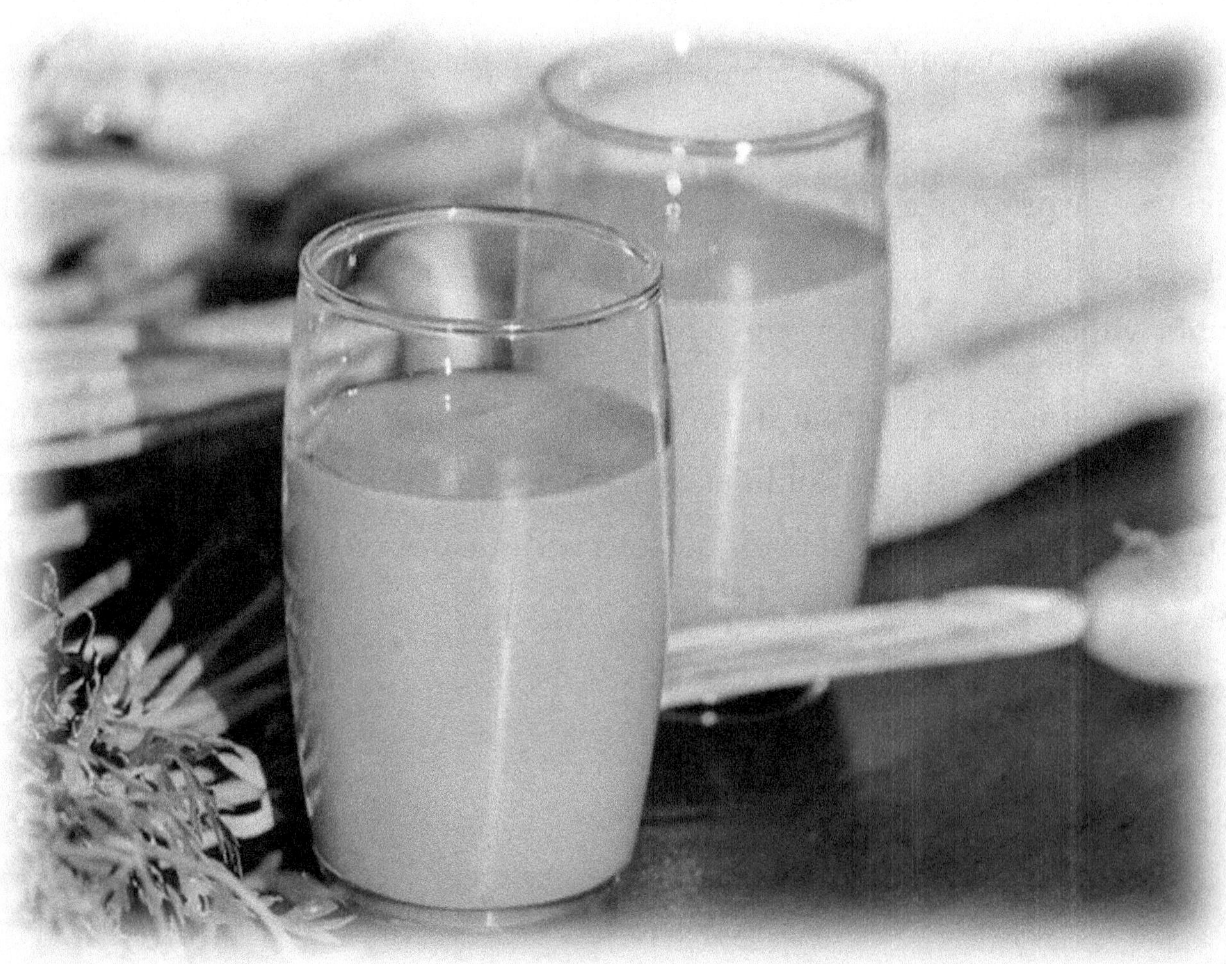

CHAPTER 1

Understanding Gastroparesis: Causes, Symptoms, and Challenges.

Gastroparesis is a chronic illness in which the stomach is unable to empty itself normally. It's a condition in which the stomach takes too long to remove its contents, which can result in a variety of symptoms and consequences that impair a person's quality of life and health.

Causes of Gastroparesis

The actual etiology of gastroparesis is generally unknown, but it has been linked to injury to the vagus nerve, which controls the digestive system. There are various things that might cause nerve damage:

- Diabetes: High blood sugar can cause chemical changes in nerves and blood vessels that transport oxygen and nutrients, including the vagus nerve.
- Surgery: Procedures involving the stomach or small intestine can mistakenly injure the vagus nerve.
- Viral Infections: Certain viruses might cause gastroparesis.
- Drugs: Some drugs, such as opioid pain relievers, might cause delayed stomach emptying.
- Other disorders that might cause gastroparesis include scleroderma, Parkinson's disease, and hypothyroidism.

Symptoms Of Gastroparesis

Symptoms range from moderate to severe, and may include:

- Nausea and Vomiting: Frequently vomiting undigested food that has remained in the stomach for hours after consumption.
- Feeling Full Quickly: The sense of being full after only a few eats.
- Abdominal Pain and Bloating: Symptoms include abdominal discomfort and edema.
- Heartburn is caused by the reflux of stomach acid into the oesophagus.
- Blood sugar fluctuations: Caused by the unexpected digestion and absorption of nutrients.
- Weight loss and malnutrition: Due to decreased food intake and nutrient absorption.

Challenges of Gastroparesis

Living with gastroparesis has various obstacles.

- Dietary Restrictions: Patients frequently need to adhere to a strict diet, avoiding high-fiber and fatty foods that are difficult to digest.
- Regular Medical Attention: Visits to healthcare providers for symptom treatment and monitoring are required.
- Emotional Stress: The chronic nature of the illness can cause anxiety and sadness.
- Nutritional Deficiencies: Difficulty maintaining a balanced diet might result in deficiencies and other health concerns.

Understanding gastroparesis is the first step toward alleviating symptoms and enhancing quality of life.

Individuals suffering from gastroparesis can nourish their bodies without creating more difficulty by carefully organizing their diet, which includes juicing.

Always consult a healthcare practitioner before making any significant modifications to your gastroparesis diet or treatment plan.

How Juicing Can Help Individuals with Gastroparesis

Juicing has developed as a therapeutic therapy for people with gastroparesis, providing a means to consume critical nutrients while reducing the discomfort associated with the illness.

Nutrient Absorption

Gastroparesis can make it difficult to absorb nutrients from solid foods because the stomach empties slowly.

Juicing removes vitamins and minerals from fruits and vegetables, making them more easily absorbed without significant digestion.

Symptom Management

Juicing minimizes the chance of worsening symptoms such as bloating, nausea, and abdominal pain by eliminating fiber, which can be difficult for gastroparesis patients to digest.

This lets people to enjoy a larger range of fruit without experiencing the discomfort that comes with eating it whole.

Hydration

Juicing can help you stay hydrated, which is important for your overall health. This is especially critical for gastroparesis patients, who may struggle to consume solid foods and require enough fluids.

Customization

Juicing enables for personalization based on personal tolerances and preferences. People with gastroparesis can create juice blends that avoid their specific trigger foods and focus on ingredients that they can tolerate well.

Enhanced Variety and Taste

A gastroparesis-friendly diet might sometimes be restricted and bland. Juicing allows you to incorporate a variety of flavors and colours into your diet, making meals more pleasurable and reducing nutritional monotony.

Convenient and portable

Juices are simple to take, especially for those who do not always have the appetite or capacity to eat larger meals. They can also be carried and consumed on the go, allowing people to keep their nutritional intake consistent throughout the day.

Supporting Overall Health

Juicing a variety of fruits and vegetables might improve general health by supplying antioxidants, phytochemicals, and enzymes that may be lacking in a restrictive gastroparesis diet.

Potential for symptom improvement.

Some people have reported improved gastroparesis symptoms after introducing juicing into their diet. While not a cure, it can be used in conjunction with other treatments to manage the illness.

Juicing can be a beneficial supplement to a gastroparesis patient's diet, providing nutritional benefits as well as respite from symptoms.

However, juicing should be approached with prudence and discussed with a healthcare practitioner to verify it is appropriate for your unique health needs.

Safety Considerations for Juicing

When it comes to juicing, especially for people who have health issues like gastroparesis, safety comes first. Here are some important safety factors to bear in mind.

- Cleanliness: Always begin with clean hands, tools, and produce. Wash fruits and vegetables thoroughly to remove bacteria and chemicals.
- Equipment safety: Always follow the manufacturer's recommendations while using juicers. Before using the juicer, make sure all pieces are properly attached, and never insert your fingers or utensils into it while it is operating.
- Avoiding Harmful Ingredients: Juicing certain fruits and vegetables, such as rhubarb leaves and citrus peels, can be poisonous or harmful. Always understand which portions are safe to juice.
- Temperature Control: If you are not going to drink the juice right away, refrigerate it to prevent bacterial growth. Juices should be taken as quickly as possible after producing them.

- Pasteurization: If you have a weaker immune system, consider using pasteurized items to lower your risk of foodborne illness. Pasteurization eliminates dangerous microorganisms without dramatically altering nutritional content.
- Allergies and Interactions: Be cautious of any dietary allergies or potential drug interactions. Some additives can reduce the efficiency of medications or trigger adverse responses.
- Nutritional Balance: Juicing should be used to supplement, rather than replace, a well-balanced diet. Make sure you obtain a range of nutrients from other foods as well.
- expert Advice: Before making any big changes to your diet, such as including juicing, contact with a healthcare expert, especially if you have gastroparesis or other health concerns.

By following these safety guidelines, you can reap the benefits of juicing while reducing any hazards.

CHAPTER 2: ESSENTIAL KITCHEN TOOLS AND EQUIPMENT

Choosing the Right Juicer

Choosing the correct juicer is critical for anyone trying to incorporate juicing into their diet, particularly those with gastroparesis. Here are some points to consider while purchasing a juicer:

- There are three primary types of juicers: centrifugal, masticating, and dual gear. Centrifugal juicers are faster and typically less expensive, but they may not handle leafy greens as well as other types. Masticating juicers, often known as slow juicers, operate at slower speeds, conserving more nutrients and are more suited to juicing a wide range of produce. Twin gear juicers are the most efficient, but they also cost the most.

- Ease of Use Consider how simple the juicer is to build, use, and clean. Some juicers have more parts and may take longer to clean, which might be a deciding factor for everyday use.

- Nutrient Retention Masticating and twin gear juicers are often better at maintaining nutrients since they run at slower speeds, decreasing heat and oxidation.

- Noise Level Centrifugal juicers are generally louder than masticating or dual gear juicers. If noise is an issue, particularly for early morning or late-night juicing, you may want to consider a quieter model.

- Space and Design Think about the size of the juicer and how much counter space it will take up. Consider how the design will blend into the overall style of your kitchen.

- Budget: Determine how much you are willing to spend. While higher-end juicers may have more features and efficiency, there are many dependable ones available at a lower price point.
- Warranty and Customer Support Check the warranty period and coverage. If you have any problems with your juicer, good customer service can be really helpful.

By taking these elements into account, you may pick a juicer that best suits your needs and lifestyle, making your juicing experience for gastroparesis treatment as effective and fun as possible.

Proper Cleaning and Maintenance

Proper cleaning and maintenance of your juicer are essential for preserving its longevity and efficacy, especially when used to treat disorders such as gastroparesis.

1. Immediate Cleaning: After each use, remove your juicer and clean all parts to avoid pulp and residue from drying and sticking, making cleaning more difficult later on and potentially harboring bacteria.

2. Use the Right Tools: Many juicers have specialized brushes for cleaning mesh strainers and filters. Use these tools to remove fibres and pulp without hurting the delicate screens.

3. Warm Soapy Water: Soak and wash any parts that are not dishwasher-safe in warm soapy water. Using a soft sponge or cloth, gently clean each component.

4. Rinse thoroughly: Use warm water to remove all soap and debris from the juicer parts. Any soap residue might alter the flavor of your juice and perhaps create health problems.

5. Allow all parts to completely dry before reassembling the juicer. This helps to avoid mold and mildew formation, which is especially important for people with gastroparesis because their digestive systems may be more sensitive.

6. Deep cleaning should be done on a regular basis, even if you clean every day. Pay close attention to the cutting blades and tiny mesh regions, since particles can build over time.

7. Check for Wear and Tear: Inspect your juicer on a regular basis for signs of wear, such as dull blades or a frayed power wire. To maintain optimal performance, replace any necessary parts.

8. When not in use, keep your juicer in a clean and dry place. Cover it to keep dust and other impurities out.

Following these measures will guarantee that your juicer stays a dependable instrument for making gastroparesis-friendly juices, thereby contributing to a safe and healthy juicing routine.

CHAPTER 3: PREPARING PRODUCE FOR JUICING.

Choosing Fresh, High-Quality Ingredients

Choosing fresh, high-quality ingredients is essential for preparing nutritious and safe juices for people with gastroparesis.

Gastroparesis necessitates cautious selection of fruits and vegetables that are unlikely to worsen symptoms. Select food that is low in fiber and easy to digest.

Choose peelable fruits with low fiber content. Good choices include:

- Peeled apples and pear.
- Bananas
- Melons.
- Papayas.
- Peaches and nectarines (canned in natural juice for diabetics)
- Mangos.

Choose veggies that can be thoroughly boiled and peeled to lower fiber content. Suitable vegetables include:

- Potatoes
- Carrots.
- Parsnips.
- Beets.
- Zucchini
- Eggplant.

When it comes to juicing, the quality of the components is more important than quantity. Fresh, ripe, and seasonal produce produces the tastiest and nutrient-dense juices.

If feasible, pick organic vegetables to reduce pesticide exposure, which is especially important for people with sensitive digestive systems. If organic produce is neither available or viable, make sure to properly wash conventional vegetables.

Choose ripe but not overripe fruits and vegetables for the best enzyme and nutrient balance. Overripe food may ferment more quickly, which could cause pain.

Proper storage and handling of your ingredients is critical. Keep your produce in a clean, cool place, and carefully wash it before juicing to remove dirt and bacteria.

Peel and remove seeds from fruits and vegetables, as they are generally high in fiber. Cut produce into small bits that will fit down your juicer's feed chute.

Rotate your foods on a regular basis to ensure that your diet contains a diverse range of nutrients. This also aids in determining which fruits or veggies you may be more sensitive to.

By carefully selecting and preparing your ingredients, you may make delicious and nutritious juices that meet the needs of your gastroparesis diet, giving critical vitamins and minerals while reducing the danger of exacerbating your symptoms.

Peeling, Chopping, and Preparation Techniques

When it comes to juicing for gastroparesis, proper peeling, chopping, and preparing skills are essential to ensure that the juice is as mild on the stomach as possible.

Peeling

- Peel fruits and vegetables to reduce fiber content, which can be difficult to digest for those with gastroparesis.
- Use a Vegetable Peeler: A decent peeler will help you remove peels quickly and safely.
- Be thorough: Remove all skin, as even tiny quantities of fiber can cause irritation.

Chopping

- Small bits: Cut vegetables into small, manageable bits that are easier to juice and less likely to clog the juicer.
- Consistent Size: Keep the pieces uniform in size to enable even juicing and nutrient extraction.
- Gentle Handling: To protect the produce's integrity, chop gently, especially if it is tender or ripe.

Prepping

- Remove seeds and cores: Seeds and cores are difficult to digest and may contain stomach-irritating substances.
- Rinse Well: After peeling, properly rinse your produce to remove any `lingering dirt or bacteria.

- Blanching: For some veggies, a quick blanch and shock (boil briefly before plunging into freezing water) can make them softer and simpler to juice.

By using these approaches, you may make juices that are not only healthy but also easy to digest for people with gastroparesis. Remember, the goal is to make juicing a pleasurable and health-promoting experience.

How to Store Produce for Maximum Freshness

Storing produce correctly is critical for preserving freshness, especially when juicing for gastroparesis. Here are some techniques to keep your fruits and veggies fresh until you're ready to juice them.

- Cool, Dry, Dark Place: Store certain veggies like onions, garlic, and hard squashes in a pantry or cupboard away from light to avoid sprouting.
- Refrigerator Crisper Drawers: To keep vegetables fresher for longer, set the humidity to high. The fridge temperature should be between 33 and 40°F.
- Don't Wash Until Ready to Use: Keep vegetables unwashed in storage to avoid spoiling. Wash them shortly before preparing to juice.
- Do Not Cut Produce Until Juicing: Cutting increases the surface area exposed to air, which might accelerate the degradation process.
- Store with airflow: For most vegetables, avoid airtight containers, since some airflow helps keep freshness.
- Separate Ethylene Producers: Certain fruits, such as bananas and apples, release ethylene gas, which can accelerate the ripening and spoiling of other products. Store them individually.

CHAPTER 4: JUICING TECHNIQUES AND TIPS.

Slow Vs. Centrifugal Juicers: Pros and Cons

When juicing for gastroparesis, the decision between slow and centrifugal juicers is important. Each variety offers advantages and disadvantages that can affect the juicing experience and the juice's acceptability for people with gastroparesis.

Slow juicers (masticating or cold-press)

Pros:

- Gentle Extraction: Slow juicers run at lower speeds, which reduces heat and oxidation. This mild approach protects more enzymes and nutrients, which is very advantageous for gastroparesis patients who require nutrient-dense juices.
- Efficiency: They extract more juice from the produce, resulting in dryer pulp. This means you receive more juice from the same number of fruits and vegetables, which can be cost-effective in the long term.
- Quiet Operation: Slow juicers are quieter, making them more user-friendly, particularly for individuals with gastroparesis.
- Versatility: Many slow juicers can handle leafy greens and wheatgrass well, making them ideal for anyone wishing to incorporate these into their gastroparesis-friendly diet.

Cons:

- Higher Cost: They are typically more expensive, which may be worth considering if you are on a tight budget.

- Longer Juicing Time: Because of the sluggish extraction process, juice is produced at a slower rate than with centrifugal machines.
- Prep Work: Because they frequently have smaller feed chutes, it takes more effort to cut fruit into smaller pieces.

Centrifugal juicers

Pros:

- Speed: Centrifugal juicers are quick to use, making them ideal for individuals who need to create juice quickly.
- Ease of Use: They are generally simple to operate and often have larger feed chutes, requiring less produce cutting.

Cons:

- Oxidation: High-speed spinning puts more air into the juice, resulting in faster nutritional oxidation and deterioration. This may not be suitable for gastroparesis patients who require the most nutritious juice possible.
- Noise: They can be quite loud, which may disturb some users.
- Less Effective with Leafy Greens: Centrifugal juicers may be ineffective at juicing leafy greens, which are a vital part of a healthy diet for gastroparesis therapy.

Slow juicers may be more suited for those with gastroparesis since they can generate higher-quality, more nutrient-dense juices.

If you value ease and speed, a centrifugal juicer may be the best option. It's critical to assess these factors based on your own demands and lifestyle.

Combining Ingredients to Optimize Flavor and Nutrition

Combining components for best flavor and nutrition in juicing, particularly for gastroparesis, requires a delicate balance. Here's how to make juice mixes that are both tasty and safe for those with this condition:

- Begin with a basis: Use a light, low-fiber basis such peeled cucumbers or melons. These offer hydration without overpowering the stomach.
- offer Flavor: Use fruits such as peeled apples or ripe bananas to offer natural sweetness without too much fiber. Berries can also be used for their flavor and antioxidant content.
- Include Nutrients: Leafy greens, such as spinach, can be added in tiny amounts to provide nutrients. If greens are excessively fibrous, consider using green vegetable juices that have been filtered to remove extra fiber.
- Use Herbs and Spices: Fresh herbs such as mint or ginger can enhance flavor and provide digestive benefits. Ginger, specifically, is recognized for its relaxing effects.
- Consider Protein and Fats: For a more balanced juice, add protein powder or a little amount of oil, such as flaxseed oil, to help with nutritional absorption and satiety.
- Experiment with Sweetness: If more sweetness is required, consider using a tiny quantity of honey or maple syrup, but be cautious with the proportions to avoid sugar overdose.
- Balance Acidity: If you can handle mild acidity, a modest squeeze of lemon or lime juice can brighten flavors. However, acidity might irritate the stomach.
- Test and adapt: Since everyone's tolerance is different, it's crucial to test out novel combinations in small doses and adapt based on your body's response.

Changing Juice Consistency for Gastroparesis

Adjusting the consistency of juice is a significant concern for people with gastroparesis since it affects how well the juice is tolerated. Here are some tips for adjusting juice consistency:

1. Straining: Using a fine mesh strainer or cheesecloth, remove any residual pulp from the juice. This can help generate a smoother and more digestible drink.

2. Dilution: If the juice is excessively thick, thin it with water or a low-fiber juice like apple or grape. This makes food easier to eat and less likely to create fullness or bloating.

3. Thickeners: For people who need a thicker consistency to control symptoms like reflux, consider adding a tiny amount of a gastroparesis-friendly thickening, such as guar gum or xanthan gum, which do not contribute considerable fiber content.

4. Temperature: Serving juice cold can help with nausea, but if cold liquids are not well-tolerated, room temperature or slightly warm juices may be more comfortable.

5. Blending: If adding items like protein powders or oils for nutritional benefit, use a blender to ensure these additions are well-absorbed without generating a gritty texture.

6. Serving Size: Begin with tiny servings to test tolerance and gradually increase as needed. Smaller portions are often easier to digest.

By carefully regulating the consistency of your juices, you may guarantee that they deliver nutritional advantages while without increasing gastroparesis symptoms. Before making any large dietary or juicing changes, always consult with a healthcare practitioner.

<u>Cucumber-Mint Cleanse</u>

Prep time: 10 minutes.

Serves: 1

Ingredients:

- One large, peeled cucumber
- One handful of fresh mint leaves.
- 1/2 cup water (optional for diluting).

Preparation:

- Rinse the cucumber and mint leaves completely.
- Peel the cucumber to minimize the fiber content.
- Juice the cucumbers and mint leaves together.
- If needed, dilute with water to achieve a lighter consistency.
- Serve cold for a refreshing cleansing.

Nutrition Information: Calories: approximately 45, fiber: less than 1 gram. Vitamin K: good source, excellent hydration.

Simple Spinach Elixir

Prep time: 10 minutes.

Serves: 1

Ingredients:

- 2 cups baby spinach, properly cleaned.
- One peeled green apple (optional if tolerated).
- 1/2 cup water (optional for diluting).

Preparation:

- Ensure the spinach is clean and free of dirt.
- Peel the green apple to remove the skin.
- Juice the spinach and green apple together.
- Dilute with water if you like a thinner consistency.
- Enjoy this nutrient-dense elixir.

Nutrition Information: Calories: ~60, fiber: <1g. Iron: Good source. Vitamins: A, C

Gentle Kale Tonic

Prep time: 10 minutes.

Serves: 1

Ingredients:

- 2 large kale leaves with stems removed.
- 1/2 peeled cucumber.
- 1/4 cup water (optional for diluting).

Preparation:

- Rinse the greens and cucumber.
- Peel the cucumber to remove excess fiber.
- Juice the kale and cucumber together.
- If you want a thinner juice, add more water.
- Use this green tonic to replenish your body.

Nutrition Information: Calories: ~50, fiber: <1g. Calcium: A good source. Antioxidants: High

Green Apple Hydration

Prep time: 10 minutes.

Serves: 1

Ingredients:

- One green apple, peeled and cored
- 1/2 peeled cucumber.
- 1/2 cup water (optional for diluting).

Preparation:

- Wash the apples and cucumbers.
- Peel both to lower their fiber content.
- Juice the apples and cucumbers together.
- Dilute with water to the desired consistency.
- This hydrated juice is ideal for a quick refresh.

Nutrition Information: Calories: approximately 70, fiber: less than 1g. Vitamin C: good source, excellent hydration.

Spinach-Cucumber Cooler

Prep time: 10 minutes.

Serves: 1

Ingredients:

- 1 cup baby spinach, washed
- One large, peeled cucumber
- 1/4 cup water (optional for diluting).

Preparation:

- Thoroughly clean the spinach leaves.
- Peel the cucumber to make it more gastroparesis-friendly.
- Juice the spinach and cucumber together.
- Add water if you prefer a thinner juice.
- Chill and serve this nice green beverage.

Nutrition Information: Calories: ~50, fiber: <1g. Vitamin K: good source, excellent hydration.

Celery & Parsley Refresher

Prep time: 10 minutes.

Serves: 1

Ingredients:

- 3 celery stalks, peeled
- One handful of fresh parsley leaves.
- 1/2 cup water (optional for diluting).

Preparation:

• Wash the celery and parsley thoroughly.

• Peel celery to lower fiber content.

• Juice the celery and parsley together.

• If needed, dilute with water to achieve a lighter consistency.

• Serve chilled for a refreshing beverage.

Nutrition Information: Calories: approximately 30; fiber: less than 1 gram. Vitamin C: good source, excellent hydration.

Baby Kale & Pear Delight

Prep time: 10 minutes.

Serves: 1

Ingredients:

- One cup of baby kale leaves.
- One ripe pear, peeled and cored
- 1/2 cup water (optional for diluting).

Preparation:

- Rinse the baby greens and pears.
- Peel the pear to remove excess fiber.
- Juice the baby greens and pear together.
- If you want a thinner juice, add more water.
- Savor this sweet and healthful treat.

Nutrition Information: Calories: about 70, Fiber: < 1 g. Vitamins A, C, and K Antioxidants: High

Lettuce Apple Soother.

Prep time: 10 minutes.

Serves: 1

Ingredients:

• 2 cups cleaned lettuce.

• One green apple, peeled and cored

• 1/2 cup water (optional for diluting).

Preparation:

- Wash the lettuce and apple thoroughly.
- Peel the apple to lower its fiber content.
- Juice the lettuce and apple together.
- Dilute with water to the desired consistency.
- This calming drink is ideal for a modest nutritional boost.

Nutrition Information: Calories: ~60, fiber: <1g. Vitamin K: good source, excellent hydration.

Green Melon Cooler

Prep time: 10 minutes.

Serves: 1

Ingredients:

- Two cups of honeydew melon, peeled and seeded
- Some fresh mint leaves.
- 1/2 cup water (optional for diluting).

Preparation:

- Wash the honeydew melon and mint leaves.
- Peel and seed the melon to keep it low in fiber.
- Juice the melon and mint together.
- Add water if you prefer a thinner consistency.
- On a warm day, serve this cool and pleasant drink.

Nutrition Information: Calories: ~60, fiber: <1g. Vitamin C: good source, excellent hydration.

Arugula & Mint Revival

Prep time: 10 minutes.

Serves: 1

Ingredients:

- 1 cup washed arugula.
- One handful of fresh mint leaves.
- 1/2 cup water (optional for diluting).

Preparation:

- Ensure the arugula and mint are clean and free of dirt.
- Juice the arugula and mint leaves together.
- Dilute with water if a lighter consistency is preferred.
- Try this spicy and refreshing juice for a fast pick-me-up.

Nutrition Information: Calories: approximately 20; fiber: less than 1 gram. Vitamin A: A good source. Hydration: excellent.

CHAPTER 6: FRUIT-BASED JUICES.

Papaya Peach Sip

Prep time: 10 minutes.

Serves: 1

Ingredients:

- 1/2 cup papaya, peeled and seeded
- One ripe peach, peeled and pitted
- 1/2 cup water (optional for diluting).

Preparation:

- Rinse the papaya and peach completely.
- Peel the papaya and remove its seeds, as well as the peach pit.
- Juice the two fruits together.
- If needed, dilute with water to achieve a lighter consistency.
- Serve this tropical drink chilled.

Nutrition Information: Calories: approximately 120, fiber: less than 1 gram. Vitamin C: Excellent source; Vitamin A: Good source.

Banana-Berry Smoothie

Prep time: 10 minutes.

Serves: 1

Ingredients:

- One ripe banana.
- 1/2 cup mixed berries (strawberries and blueberries), fresh or frozen.
- 1/2 cup water or lactose-free milk (optional for diluting).

Preparation:

- Peel the banana.
- Thaw any frozen berries before using them.
- Blend the banana and berries until smooth.
- If you like a thinner consistency, use water or lactose-free milk.
- Savor this berry-rich smoothie.

Nutrition Information: Calories: approximately 150, fiber: less than 2g. Vitamin C: A good source. Antioxidants: High

Melon Grape Medley.

Prep time: 10 minutes.

Serves: 1

Ingredients:

- 1 cup honeydew melons, peeled and seeded
- 1/2 cup seedless grapes, rinsed
- 1/2 cup water (optional for diluting).

Preparation:

- Wash the melon and grapes thoroughly.
- Peel and seed the watermelon.
- Juice the melon and grapes together.
- Dilute with water for a thinner consistency.
- Chill this combination of melon and grapes.

Nutrition Information: Calories: ~100, fiber: <1g. Vitamin C: good source, excellent hydration.

<u>Kiwi Strawberry Splash.</u>

Prep time: 10 minutes.

Serves: 1

Ingredients:

- Two ripe, peeled kiwis
- 1/2 cup hulled strawberries.
- 1/2 cup water (optional for diluting).

Preparation:

- Wash the kiwis and strawberries.
- Peel kiwis and hull strawberries.
- Juice the two fruits together.
- Add water if a lighter consistency is desired.
- Serve this refreshing kiwi and strawberry smoothie chilled.

Nutrition Information: Calories: ~90, fiber: <2g. Vitamin C: excellent source; Vitamin K: good source.

Mango Nectarine Delight.

Prep time: 10 minutes.

Serves: 1

Ingredients:

- One ripe mango, peeled and pitted
- One ripe nectarine, peeled and pitted
- 1/2 cup water (optional for diluting).

Preparation:

- Rinse the mango and nectarine completely.
- Peel and remove the pits from both fruits.
- Juice the mangoes and nectarine together.
- If preferred, dilute with water to make a lighter drink.
- Enjoy this wonderful mango and nectarine combination.

Nutrition Information: Calories: approximately 150, fiber: less than 2g. Vitamin C: Excellent source; Vitamin A: Good source.

Cantaloupe and Honeydew Melody

Prep time: 10 minutes.

Serves: 1

Ingredients:

- 1/2 cup cantaloupe, peeled and seeded
- 1/2 cup honeydew melon, peeled and seeded
- 1/2 cup water (optional for diluting).

Preparation:

- Thoroughly wash both melons.
- Peel and remove seeds from cantaloupe and honeydew.
- Juice both melons simultaneously.
- If needed, dilute with water to achieve a lighter consistency.
- Serve this chilled melody of melons.

Nutrition Information: Calories: ~100, fiber: <1g. Vitamin C: Excellent source; Vitamin A: Good source.

Watermelon Mint Juice

Prep time: 10 minutes.

Serves: 1

Ingredients:

- 2 cups watermelon, peeled and seeded
- Some fresh mint leaves.
- 1/2 cup water (optional for diluting).

Preparation:

- Wash the watermelon and mint leaves.
- Peel and seed a watermelon.
- Juice the watermelon and mint together.
- Dilute with water for a thinner consistency.
- Drink this delicious beverage on a hot day.

Nutrition Information: Calories: ~80, fiber: <1g. Vitamin C: good source, excellent hydration.

Blueberry Coconut Swirl.

Prep time: 10 minutes.

Serves: 1

Ingredients:

- 1/2 cup blueberries (fresh or frozen)
- One-half cup coconut water
- 1/2 cup water (optional for diluting).

Preparation:

- Make care to defrost frozen blueberries before using them.
- Blend the blueberries and coconut water until smooth.
- Add water if a lighter consistency is desired.
- Serve this tropical swirl cold for a hydrating drink.

Nutrition Information: Calories: ~50, fiber: <1g. Antioxidants: High. Electrolytes: Good source.

Apple Carrot Blend

Prep time: 10 minutes.

Serves: 1

Ingredients:

- One green apple, peeled and cored
- Two carrots, peeled
- 1/2 cup water (optional for diluting).

Preparation:

- Wash the apples and carrots.
- Peel apples and carrots to minimize fiber content.
- Juice the apples and carrots together.
- Dilute with water to the desired consistency.
- This blend is ideal for a sweet, earthy juice.

Nutrition Information: Calories: approximately 90, fiber: less than 1 gram.
Vitamin A: Excellent source; Vitamin C: Good source.

Peach Ginger Brew.

Prep time: 10 minutes.

Serves: 1

Ingredients:

- One ripe peach, peeled and pitted
- 1 inch piece of peeled ginger
- 1/2 cup water (optional for diluting).

Preparation:

- Wash the peach and ginger.
- Peel the peaches and ginger.
- Juice the peach and ginger together.
- Add water if a lighter consistency is desired.
- Serve this warming beverage to calm and refresh.

Nutrition Information: Calories: about 60, Fiber: < 1 g. Gingerol (from ginger): A good source. Vitamin C: Good source.

CHAPTER 7: VEGETABLE-BASED JUICES

Carrot Celery Calm.

Prep time: 10 minutes.

Serves: 1

Ingredients:

- Two large, peeled carrots
- Two celery stalks, peeled

Preparation:

- Wash the carrots and celery thoroughly.
- Peel the vegetables to lower their fiber content.
- Juice the carrot and celery together.
- Serve immediately for a calming drink.

Nutrition Information: Calories: approximately 70, fiber: less than 1g. Vitamin A: Excellent source; Vitamin K: Good source.

Zucchini And Cucumber Cooler

Prep time: 10 minutes.

Serves: 1

Ingredients:

- One medium zucchini, peeled
- 1/2 big, peeled cucumber.

Preparation:

- Wash the zucchini and cucumber.
- Peel the vegetables to keep them low in fiber.
- Juice the zucchini and cucumber together.
- Chill and serve this refreshing beverage.

Nutrition Information: Calories: ~50, fiber: <1g. Vitamin C: good source, excellent hydration.

Beetroot Cucumber Cure

Prep time: 10 minutes.

Serves: 1

Ingredients:

- One small, peeled beetroot
- 1/2 cucumber, peeled.

Preparation:

- Wash the beetroot and cucumber.
- Peel vegetables to reduce fiber content.
- Juice the beets and cucumber together.
- Serve this nutrient-dense juice for a health boost.

Nutrition Information: Calories: ~60, fiber: <1g, folate: good supply, potassium: good source.

Squash Bell Pepper Brew

Prep time: 10 minutes.

Serves: 1

Ingredients:

- 1 cup butternut squash (peeled and seeded)
- 1/2 red bell pepper with seeds removed

Preparation:

- Wash the squash and bell pepper.
- Peel and remove the squash seeds.
- Juice the squash and bell pepper together.
- Indulge in this sweet and Savory mix.

Nutrition Information: Calories: ~80, fiber: <1g. Vitamin A is an excellent source, as is vitamin C.

Radish Cabbage Relief

Prep time: 10 minutes.

Serves: 1

Ingredients:

- 1/2 cup cleaned radishes.
- 1 cup cleaned green cabbage.

Preparation:

- Ensure that the radishes and cabbage are clean.
- Juice the radishes and cabbage together.
- Serve this moderate juice to alleviate intestinal discomfort.

Nutrition Information: Calories: approximately 40, fiber: less than 1 gram. Vitamin C: A good source. Antioxidants: High

Sweet Potato Broth

Prep time: 15 minutes.

Serves: 1

Ingredients:

- One medium sweet potato, peeled
- 1/2 teaspoon ground cinnamon (optional).

Preparation:

- Wash and peel the sweet potatoes.
- Cut into small chunks that will fit in your juicer.
- Squeeze the sweet potato.
- Warm the juice on the heat, then add cinnamon if desired.
- Serve this warm broth to calm your tummy.

Nutrition Information: Calories: ~100, fiber: <1g. Vitamin A is an excellent source. Potassium: A good source.

Pumpkin Carrot Comfort

Prep time: 15 minutes.

Serves: 1

Ingredients:

- 1 cup pumpkin, peeled and seeded
- Two large, peeled carrots

Preparation:

- Wash the pumpkin and carrots.
- Peel and chop into bits.
- Juice the pumpkin and carrots together.
- This comfortable blend can be served warm or as is.

Nutrition Information: Calories: ~80, fiber: <1g. Vitamin A: Excellent source; Vitamin C: Good source.

Asparagus With Spinach Tonic

Prep time: 15 minutes.

Serves: 1

Ingredients:

- 5 asparagus spears (trimmed)
- 1 cup cleaned spinach.

Preparation:

- Wash the asparagus and spinach thoroughly.
- Juice the asparagus and spinach together.
- To reap the digestion advantages, serve this green tonic immediately.

Nutrition Information: Calories: approximately 40, fiber: less than 1 gram. Folate is a good source Vitamins A, C, and K

Eggplant Parsley Potion

Prep time: 15 minutes.

Serves: 1

Ingredients:

- 1/2 medium eggplant, peeled.
- One handful of fresh parsley leaves.

Preparation:

- Wash and peel the eggplant.
- Juice the eggplant and parsley together.
- This one-of-a-kind potion can be served cold or at room temperature.

Nutrition Information: Calories: ~35, fiber: <1g. Antioxidants: High. Vitamin B: Good source.

Turnip and Fennel Fusion

Prep time: 15 minutes.

Serves: 1

Ingredients:

- One medium turnip, peeled
- 1/2 fennel bulb.

Preparation:

- Wash and peel the turnips.
- Clean the fennel bulb and cut it into pieces to fit your juicer.
- Juice the turnips and fennel together.
- Serve this combination as a pleasant and digestion-friendly beverage.

Nutrition Information: Calories: ~50, fiber: <1g. Manganese and Vitamin C are both good sources.

CHAPTER 8: COMBINATION JUICES.

Spinach Carrot Combo

Prep time: 10 minutes.

Serves: 1

Ingredients:

- 1 cup cleaned spinach.
- Two carrots, peeled

Preparation:

- Wash the spinach thoroughly.
- Peel the carrots to minimize the fiber content.
- Juice the spinach and carrots together.
- Serve this combination for a nutrient-dense beverage.

Nutrition Information: Calories: approximately 70, fiber: less than 1g. Vitamin A: Excellent source; Vitamin C: Good source.

Kale-Apple Fusion

Prep time: 10 minutes.

Serves: 1

Ingredients:

- 1 cup kale (stems removed)
- One green apple, peeled and cored

Preparation:

- Rinse the kale leaves.
- Peel and core the apples.
- Juice the greens and apple together.
- Enjoy this blend for a vitamin-rich refreshment.

Nutrition Information: Calories: around 80, fiber: less than 1g, vitamins: A, C, and K. Calcium: A good source.

Spinach, Apple, and Ginger Green Machine

Prep time: 10 minutes.

Serves: 1

Ingredients:

- 1 cup cleaned spinach.
- One green apple, peeled and cored
- 1 inch piece of peeled ginger

Preparation:

- Clean the spinach and apple.
- Peel and core the apple; peel the ginger.
- Juice all of the ingredients together.
- Drink this green machine as a digestion help.

Nutrition Information: Calories: approximately 90, fiber: less than 1 gram. Gingerol: A good source. Vitamins: A, C

Cucumber Melon Mixture

Prep time: 10 minutes.

Serves: 1

Ingredients:

- 1/2 cucumber, peeled.
- 2 cups honeydew melons, peeled and seeded

Preparation:

- Wash the cucumbers and honeydew melon.
- Peel and seed the melon; peel the cucumber.
- Juice the cucumber and melon together.
- Serve chilled for a hydrating effect.

Nutrition Information: Calories: ~100, fiber: <1g. Vitamin C: good source, excellent hydration.

Carrot Apple Ginger

Prep time: 10 minutes.

Serves: 1

Ingredients:

- Two carrots, peeled
- One green apple, peeled and cored
- 1 inch piece of peeled ginger

Preparation:

- Wash the carrots, apples, and ginger.
- Peel all ingredients to reduce fiber.
- Juice the carrots, apples, and ginger together.
- Drink this spicy-sweet juice anytime of day.

Nutrition Information: Calories: approximately 110, fiber: less than 1g. Vitamin A: Excellent source; Vitamin C: Good source.

Green Tea Citrus Infusion

Prep time: 15 minutes.

Serves: 1

Ingredients:

- 1 cup of brewed and chilled green tea
- One-half peeled orange
- Some fresh mint leaves.

Preparation:

- Brew the green tea and let it cool.
- Peel the orange to lower the fiber content.
- Juice the peeled oranges and mint leaves.
- Mix the juice with the green tea.
- Keep this infusion cold for a refreshing boost.

Nutrition Information: Calories: ~60, fiber: <1g. Vitamin C: A good source.
Antioxidants: High

Avocado Berry Blend.

Prep time: 10 minutes.

Serves: 1

Ingredients:

- One-half ripe avocado
- 1/2 cup mixed berries (strawberries and blueberries), fresh or frozen.
- 1/2 cup water or lactose-free milk (optional for diluting).

Preparation:

- Scoop out the avocado flesh.
- Thaw any frozen berries before using them.
- Blend the avocado and berries until smooth.
- If you like a thinner consistency, use water or lactose-free milk.
- Savor this creamy mix.

Nutrition Information: Calories: approximately 200, fiber: less than 2g. A good source of healthy fats and vitamin E.

Pumpkin Apple Spice

Prep time: 15 minutes.

Serves: 1

Ingredients:

- 1 cup pumpkin, peeled and seeded
- One green apple, peeled and cored
- One pinch of ground cinnamon (optional)

Preparation:

- Wash the pumpkin and apple.
- Peel and chop into bits.
- Juice the pumpkin and apple together.
- Add a pinch of cinnamon if preferred.
- Serve this spicy juice as a soothing treat.

Nutrition Information: Calories: approximately 90, fiber: less than 1 gram. Vitamin A: Excellent source; Vitamin C: Good source.

Fennel, Pear and Ginger Digestive Aid

Prep time: 15 minutes.

Serves: 1

Ingredients:

- 1/2 fennel bulb.
- One ripe pear, peeled and cored
- 1 inch piece of peeled ginger

Preparation:

- Wash the fennel, pear, and ginger.
- Peel the pears and ginger.
- Juice the fennel, pear, and ginger together.
- Use this digestive aid to ease your stomach.

Nutrition Information: Calories: ~100, fiber: <1g. Gingerol: A good source. Vitamins C and K

Arugula, Grapefruit and Mint Reviver

Prep time: 15 minutes.

Serves: 1

Ingredients:

- 1 cup washed arugula.
- 1/2 grapefruit, peeled and seeded.
- One handful of fresh mint leaves.

Preparation:

- Ensure the arugula is clean and free of dirt.
- Peel the grapefruit to remove the peel and seeds.
- Juice the arugula, grapefruit, and mint together.
- Savor this energizing juice blend.

Nutrition Information: Calories: approximately 70, fiber: less than 1g.

Vitamin C: Excellent source; Vitamin A: Good source.

Almond Milk and Chia Seed Mix

Prep time: 10 minutes.

Serves: 1

Ingredients:

- One cup unsweetened almond milk.
- One spoonful of chia seeds.

Preparation:

- Pour almond milk into a glass.
- Add the chia seeds and stir thoroughly.
- Allow the mixture to sit for 5 minutes so that the chia seeds can swell and soften.
- Stir again before drinking to ensure a smooth consistency.

Nutrition Information: Calories: ~60, Fiber: <1g, Omega-3 Fatty Acids: Good source, Calcium: Good source.

Spirulina Cucumber Splash

Prep time: 10 minutes.

Serves: 1

Ingredients:

- 1/2 cucumber, peeled.
- One teaspoon of spirulina powder.
- One cup of water.

Preparation:

- Squeeze the peeled cucumber.
- Stir in the spirulina powder until completely dissolved.
- Dilute the mixture with water to taste.
- Serve this nutrient-rich splash cold.

Nutrition Information: Calories: approximately 30; fiber: less than 1 gram. Protein: A good source. Vitamins A and B12

Aloe Vera Apple Elixir.

Prep time: 10 minutes.

Serves: 1

Ingredients:

- 1/2 cup of aloe vera juice.
- One green apple, peeled and cored

Preparation:

- Juice a peeled and cored apple.
- Mix the apple juice and aloe vera liquid.
- Serve immediately as a calming elixir.

Nutrition Information: Calories: ~80, fiber: <1g. Vitamin C: good source, excellent hydration.

Coconut Water Electrolyte

Prep time: 5 minutes.

Serves: 1

Ingredients:

- One cup of coconut water.
- A squeeze of fresh lime juice (optional).

Preparation:

- Transfer the coconut water to a glass.
- For more flavor, add a squeeze of lime juice.
- Stir thoroughly and enjoy this hydrating beverage.

Nutrition Information: Calories: approximately 45, fiber: less than 1 gram. Potassium: An excellent source. Electrolytes: High.

Turmeric Carrot Shot

Prep time: 10 minutes.

Serves: 1

Ingredients:

- Two large, peeled carrots
- 1/2 teaspoon of turmeric powder.
- 1/2 cup of water (optional for diluting).

Preparation:

- Juice the peeled carrots.
- Stir in the turmeric powder until thoroughly incorporated.
- Dilute with water if you prefer a less concentrated shot.
- Give this anti-inflammatory shot as a health boost.

Nutrition Information: Calories: approximately 70, fiber: less than 1g. Vitamin A: Excellent source; Curcumin: Good source.

<u>Ginger Beet Concoction</u>

Prep time: 10 minutes.

Serves: 1

Ingredients:

- One small, peeled beet
- 1 inch piece of peeled ginger

Preparation:

- Wash and peel the beets and ginger.
- Juice both ingredients together.
- Serve this combination for its anti-inflammatory properties.

Nutrition Information: Calories: ~35, fiber: <1g. Vitamin C: A good source. Antioxidants: High

Broccoli Apple Essence

Prep time: 10 minutes.

Serves: 1

Ingredients:

- 1 cup broccoli with stems removed.
- One green apple, peeled and cored

Preparation:

- Rinse the broccoli and apples.
- Peel and core the apples.
- Juice the broccoli and apple together.
- Drink this essence for a vitamin-rich beverage.

Nutrition Information: Calories: ~60, fiber: <1g. Vitamin C: excellent source; Vitamin K: good source.

Kale Spinach Booster

Prep time: 10 minutes.

Serves: 1

Ingredients:

- 1 cup kale (stems removed)
- 1 cup cleaned spinach.

Preparation:

- Wash the kale and spinach well.
- Juice the kale and spinach together.
- Drink this booster to supplement your daily greens intake.

Nutrition Information: Calories: ~50, fiber: <1g. Vitamins A, C, and K Iron: good source.

Wheatgrass And Aloe Vera Shot

Prep time: 5 minutes.

Serves: 1

Ingredients:

- One ounce of wheatgrass juice.
- One ounce of aloe vera juice.

Preparation:

- Combine the wheatgrass juice and aloe vera juice together.
- Take this shot on an empty stomach to maximize absorption.

Nutrition Information: Calories: ~15; Fiber: 0g. Chlorophyll: Good supply; Enzymes: High.

Maca Root and Carrot Energy Boost

Prep time: 10 minutes.

Serves: 1

Ingredients:

- Two large, peeled carrots
- One teaspoon of maca powder.

Preparation:

- Wash and peel the carrots.
- Juice the carrots.
- Stir in the maca powder until thoroughly incorporated.
- Enjoy this energy boost, particularly in the morning.

Nutrition Information: Calories: approximately 70, fiber: less than 1g. Vitamin A: Excellent source; adaptogens: Good source.

<u>30-Day Juicing Meal Plan</u>

Week One: Introduction to Juicing

- Day 1: Cucumber Mint Cleanse
- Day 2: Simple Spinach Elixir.
- Day 3: Gentle Kale Tonic.
- Day 4: Green Apple Hydration
- Day 5: Spinach and Cucumber Cooler.
- Day 6: Celery Parsley Refresher.
- Day 7: Baby Kale with Pear Delight

Week Two: Exploring Flavors

- Day 8: Lettuce, Apple Soother
- Day 9: Green Melon Cooler.
- Day 10: Arugula and Mint Revival.
- Day 11: Papaya Peach Sip.
- Day 12 - Banana Berry Smoothie
- Day 13: Melon Grape Medley.
- Day 14 - Kiwi Strawberry Splash

Week Three: Vegetable Ventures

- Day 15 - Mango Nectarine Delight
- Day 16: Cantaloupe with Honeydew Melody
- Day 17: Watermelon-Mint Juice
- Day 18 - Blueberry Coconut Swirl
- Day 19 - Apple Carrot Blend
- Day 20 - Peach Ginger Brew
- Day 21: Carrot Celery Calm.

Week Four: Combination Creations.

- Day 22: Zucchini and cucumber cooler.
- Day 23: Beetroot-Cucumber Cure
- Day 24: Squash Bell Pepper Brew.
- Day 25: Radish Cabbage Relief.
- Day 26 - Sweet Potato Broth
- Day 27: Pumpkin Carrot Comfort.
- Day 28: Asparagus and Spinach Tonic

Week Five: Nutrient Boosters

- Day 29 - Eggplant Parsley Potion
- Day 30: Turnip and Fennel Fusion.

Remember to introduce these juices gradually, beginning with smaller amounts, to ensure that they are well accepted.

Always consult a healthcare practitioner before beginning any new dietary plan, especially if you have a disease like gastroparesis.

- **What is gastroparesis, and why is juicing beneficial?** Gastroparesis occurs when the stomach is unable to empty itself normally. Juicing is recommended because it can deliver critical nutrients while being easier to digest, as it removes the majority of the fiber that might aggravate symptoms

- **Can I juice any type of fruit or vegetable if I have gastroparesis?** If you have gastroparesis, you should avoid juicing certain fruits and vegetables. It's recommended to choose low-fiber options and avoid those that are high in fiber that may cause bloating and discomfort.

- **Is there any difference between juicing and blending for gastroparesis?** Yes, juicing removes the majority of the fiber, making it easier on your digestive system, but blending preserves all of the fiber. For gastroparesis, juicing is often more appropriate than blending

- **How can I begin juicing if I have gastroparesis?** Begin cautiously, with little amounts of juice, to watch how your body responds. Gradually increase the amount as tolerated. To lower fiber content, fruits and vegetables should be peeled and seeds removed.

- **Can juicing replace my meals?** Juicing should be used to supplement, not replace, meals. It is crucial to keep a balanced diet and ensure that you obtain enough protein and healthy fats from other sources.

- **Are there any nutritional problems to juicing?** Because juicing primarily delivers carbohydrates, it is critical to ensure that you are also getting enough protein and fat. Consider adding a protein source or a small bit of oil to your juices if necessary.

- **What are some juice recipes that are good for gastroparesis?** Some gastroparesis-friendly juice recipes include the Cucumber Mint Cleanse,

Simple Spinach Elixir, and Carrot Celery Calm, which are made with ingredients that are commonly accepted.

- **How frequently should I consume juice?** This varies by person. Some people benefit from juicing on a regular basis, while others find that juicing a few times per week suffices. Listen to your body and modify accordingly.

- **Can juicing exacerbate gastroparesis symptoms?** If done incorrectly, juicing might exacerbate symptoms. It's critical to use the appropriate components and avoid drinking too much juice at once. Always consult with a healthcare practitioner before beginning a juicing plan.

- **Should I use organic veggies when juicing?** Organic vegetables can reduce pesticide exposure, which is particularly essential for people with sensitive digestive systems. However, if organic produce is not available, be sure to properly wash conventional produce.

CONCLUSION

As we conclude this journey through "Juicing Recipes for Gastroparesis," I hope you have gained a sense of strength and a treasure trove of recipes to help you on your wellness path.

This book was written with the purpose of adding taste and nourishment to your life, despite the difficulties that gastroparesis offers.

Your experiences, insights, and feedback are extremely valuable. If this book has provided any relief, joy, or diversity in your diet, I would appreciate it if you could share your opinions.

Positive evaluations not only brighten the emotions of those who contributed to this book, but they help direct others down similar routes to find these resources. Please feel free to post a review or contact us with feedback—your voice is important.

Remember that you are not alone on this walk. Each sip of juice helps to manage your symptoms and nourish your body. It's a journey of small steps and large strides, and each day is an opportunity to prioritize your health and well-being.

May these dishes serve as a daily reminder that with a little imagination and care, you may enjoy great flavors while also meeting your body's nutritional demands. Here's to achieving balance, one juice at a time. Cheers to your health and happiness!

Thank you for making this book part of your gastroparesis experience.